Hey there

Veterinarian!

Are you concerned that you may be making serious mistakes when managing your veterinary practice?

As a veterinary practice owner, you are responsible for making numerous financial decisions each week, including accounting, taxes, payroll, banking, and more.

It can be challenging to determine the best course of action and make sound decisions that will benefit your business.

We speak with veterinarians throughout the United States every week who are exceptional at providing top-quality patient care but struggle with the business side of their practice.

If this sounds familiar, rest assured that it's not your fault.

As a veterinarian, you have devoted over 10,000 hours to perfecting your craft and delivering exceptional care to your patients.

However, you may have received limited education and training on how to grow a profitable business.

Through our research, we've found that more than 90% of veterinary practice owners make 10 common financial mistakes when running their businesses.

The worst part is that even a single mistake can cause you to work harder than necessary and earn far less profit than you should.

Fortunately, all of these mistakes can be corrected with the right guidance, saving you valuable time and thousands of dollars.

In this guide, we'll discuss the ten most significant financial mistakes made by veterinarians and provide you with actionable solutions that you can implement immediately.

So let's go over each of the 10 biggest financial mistakes veterinarians make and what you can do to fix them today

#01 Pain Point

Not Properly Compensating Employees To Retain Talent Long Term

JENNIFER KINDRED

Pain Point #01

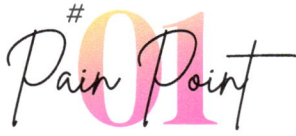

Not Properly Compensating Employees To Retain Talent Long Term

One of the most significant and persistent issues in the veterinary industry is finding, hiring, and retaining high-quality staff. In this section, we'll explore the staffing challenges clinics face, why they occur, and potential solutions.

The veterinary field demands capable staff with medical knowledge and compassion for animals. But competition is fierce for talent. Specialized training requirements limit the pool of qualified candidates.

Turnover is high due to burnout. Wages often can't match offers from human medicine. This produces constant staff shortages, from veterinary technicians to associate veterinarians.

The Importance of Fostering Teamwork

Given the complex nature of veterinary care, a cohesive team is crucial for delivering high-quality medicine. Make teamwork a priority through:

- ✔ Regular staff meetings to align on practice goals, issues, and feedback. Celebrate successes together!

- ✔ Cross-training employees in different roles to build empathy and support. Let techs shadow reception or assist with inventory.

- ✔ Team-building activities like offsite retreats, lunches, and community service projects to connect personally.

- ✔ Shared incentives like bonuses when the entire practice meets revenue goals. Foster collective success.

Pain Point #01

Not Properly Compensating Employees To Retain Talent Long Term

✔️ Dissolve cliques or "us vs. them" mentalities between departments through shared wins.

✔️ Ensure staff feel valued by leadership regardless of their role. Seek input from all levels.

With turnover rates topping 25%, investing in team culture and cohesion brings big returns through engagement, morale, and tenure.

Hiring Associate Vets

Hiring associate vets is especially problematic for veterinary practice owners.

Most new grads have large student debt burdens, so salary and compensation are key factors in job decisions. This gives corporate consolidation groups advantages in recruitment with signing bonuses and higher base salaries. Traditional private practices struggle to compete on base pay alone.

When hiring associate vets, avoid overpaying with inflated salaries that hurt profitability. Pay structures based on production incentives help level the playing field. Compensation packages that include a lower base salary plus commissions on production or procedures performed reward productivity.

Associates earn based on their hard work while the practice benefits from the revenue generated. This aligns incentives between the business and vets.

Implementing Effective Compensation Models

The pros and cons of various pay models for associates should be carefully considered.

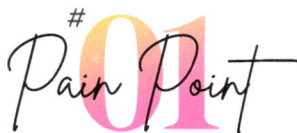

Not Properly Compensating Employees To Retain Talent Long Term

For example, pay associates $80,000 - $100,000 in base salary based on experience and credentials. Then, add quarterly commissions of 10% - 20% on production exceeding a set threshold. Structure tiers based on production growth.

Hiring Associate Vets

If the threshold is $250,000 per quarter and the vet produces $300,000, pay a 15% commission on the $50,000 above the threshold. This equals $7,500 extra for the quarter on top of base pay.

Set realistic production targets based on the practice's client load and capacity. Pay higher commission rates for higher production tiers to incentivize growth.

Make sure associate contracts spell out compensation details clearly. Track production daily and share reports with vets so they know their progress toward bonuses. This motivates them to maximize care quality and efficiency in order to increase their earnings.

Strategies for Onboarding, Training, and Retention

Effective onboarding and training establish culture and expectations. Clear policies and procedures manuals cover best practices. Quality of life incentives like work flexibility address burnout. Internal advancement opportunities encourage retention. Loan forgiveness programs for vets in high-need areas are emerging.

In the end, there are no quick fixes but continuously improving recruitment, compensation, development, and retention is key. Proactively managing staffing and compensation enables your practice to deliver exceptional animal care.

#02 *Pain Point*

Failing To Monitor Equipment Costs To Protect Profitability

JENNIFER KINDRED

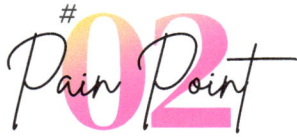

Failing To Monitor Equipment Costs To Protect Profitability

Rising operating costs are a constant challenge for veterinary practices. Equipment, supplies, drugs, staff, insurance, leases, and other overhead expenses continue increasing faster than revenue growth in most practices. This steadily compresses profit margins if costs are not effectively managed.

Some major factors driving rising veterinary costs include:

Veterinary Clinic Equipment Costs

Digital X-ray machines, dental machines, surgical lasers, and other technology have high capital costs. Maintenance and upgrades are also expensive.

Here is a breakdown of the costs associated with veterinary equipment in a veterinary practice:

Digital X-Ray Machines

- Digital X-ray machines involve a significant upfront investment, with basic units starting at around $15,000 but high-end systems costing over $100,000.

- There are ongoing costs for maintenance contracts, software updates, data storage/archiving, and periodic replacement of components like detectors. These can add up to thousands per year.

- Image quality is dependent on the system, with more expensive digital radiography units producing finer detail/resolution.

Failing To Monitor Equipment Costs To Protect Profitability

✔ Savings come from eliminating film and chemical processing costs, though digital exam workflow takes time to optimize.

Dental Machines

✔ Basic ultrasonic dental scalers start around $2,000 but more advanced piezo units run $7,000-$10,000.

✔ Dental X-ray sensors range from $3,000-$7,000. Digital dental radiograph units are $15,000+.

✔ Handpieces, burs, and other dental consumables must be continually replenished.

✔ Dental machine maintenance can exceed $2,000 annually between handpiece repairs, tubing replacement, etc.

Surgical Lasers

✔ Surgical diode lasers start around $3,000 but more powerful units run $12,000-$18,000.

✔ Laser fibers range from $100-$300 per tip and need frequent replacing.

✔ Lasers require regular calibration and maintenance to keep performing well, at a cost of ~$500/year.

✔ There are consumable costs for drapes, eyewear, etc. to maintain a sterile surgical environment.

Pain Point #02

Failing To Monitor Equipment Costs To Protect Profitability

Other Equipment

- ✔ Monitoring equipment like blood pressure monitors ($1,500+) and pulse oximeters ($500-$1,500) carry consumable costs for probes.

- ✔ Anesthesia machines ($10,000+) require regular maintenance for optimal performance and safety.

- ✔ Exam room consumables like tables, microscopes, and scales need eventual replacement too.

The high upfront investment, ongoing maintenance expenses, and continual consumable costs make veterinary equipment a significant long-term line item for any practice. Careful budgeting and equipment choices are important for managing these costs.

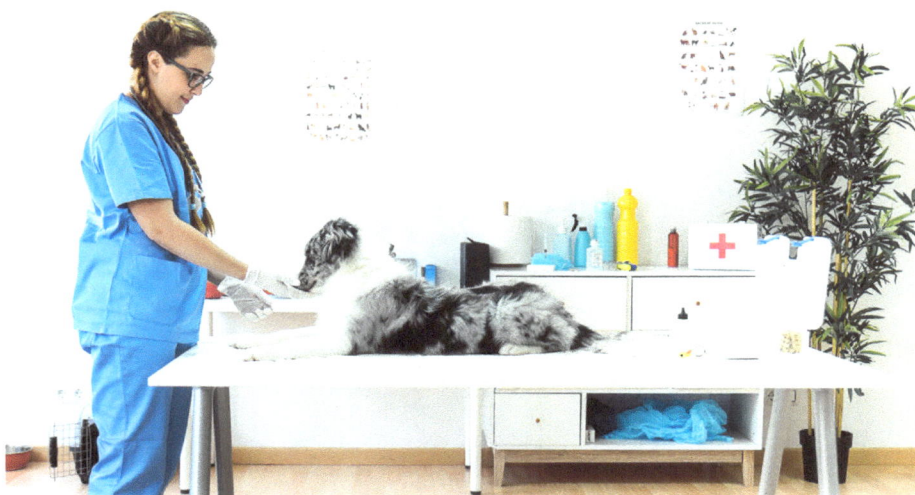

#03 Pain Point

Failing To Manage Inventory Costs To Prevent Low Profit Margins

JENNIFER KINDRED

#03 Pain Point

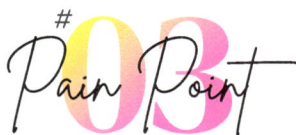

Failing To Manage Inventory Costs To Prevent Low Profit Margins

The Importance of Inventory Management

Having too much or too little inventory negatively affects your practice's finances. Excess inventory means cash flow is tied up in unused products that often expire. Insufficient inventory results in frequent ordering at higher rush costs to meet demand.

Pharmaceutical Costs and Inventory

Prescription medications make up 20-30% of the overhead for a typical veterinary practice, including the cost of maintaining an inventory of commonly used drugs. Branded drugs still under patent protection tend to be expensive, with prices increasing well above inflation annually.

Some medications like Proheart for heartworm have even doubled in price over the past decade. Generic drugs can provide some savings of 20-50% compared to branded equivalents, though availability lags behind the human market.

Best Practices for Inventory Management

Careful inventory management is crucial for minimizing waste and loss. Tracking usage over time, factoring in seasonal demand spikes, monitoring expiration dates, and avoiding overstocking with judicious reordering enables practices to limit throwaways.

Losses from inadequate inventory controls or staff errors are estimated at 0.5-3%. This includes disposal of expired drugs, breakage, incorrect charges, and potential staff theft. Diversion of prescription medications to human abuse is an emerging concern requiring tightened controls.

Pain Point #03

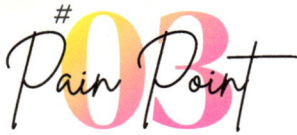

Failing To Manage Inventory Costs To Prevent Low Profit Margins

Tips to Optimize Inventory:

✔ Track item usage over time to accurately forecast demand. Factor in seasonal fluctuations. For example, heartworm medication sales spike in summer.

✔ Place bulk orders for non-perishables to get volume discounts. But don't overstock more than quarterly demand. Overordering ties up cash.

✔ Closely monitor expiration dates, especially for perishable items. Log dates when stock arrives. Pull short-dated inventory forward to minimize write-offs.

✔ Use inventory management software to automate reordering, provide real-time stock-level visibility, and trigger alerts for low items. Optimize reorder points and order quantities.

✔ Standardize supply ordering protocols and centralize purchasing to one trained manager. Enforce approval processes. Set par levels.

✔ Catalog all inventory into the system during a monthly physical count. This verifies actual stock and helps identify shrinkage issues.

With diligent purchasing, tracking, and staff training on proper procedures, veterinary practices can better control pharmaceutical overhead, minimize waste from expiration or breakage, and prevent loss from mishandling or diversion.

Optimized inventory management is essential for financial health. With a data-driven approach, you can fine-tune inventory to precisely meet clinical demand while minimizing waste and cost. For example, one clinic cut expired drug write-offs 68% annually using better monitoring and reordering processes. Regular cycle counts also improved unit accuracy.

Pain Point

#04

Failing To Utilize Industry-Specific Strategies To Optimize Cash Flow

JENNIFER KINDRED

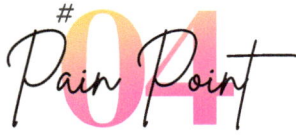

Failing To Utilize Industry-Specific Strategies To Optimize Cash Flow

The Value of Vendor Contracts

Veterinary practices often miss out on big cost savings by not utilizing purchasing contracts with vendors and suppliers. Here's how to capitalize on contracts.

Veterinary cooperatives like VetNetwork, MWI, and HealthyPaws negotiate discounted group purchasing contracts for supplies, services, pharmaceuticals, and more. This removes the hassle of sourcing your own deals.

Contracts guarantee you the lowest prices. For example, VetNetwork members get 50% off Crocs shoes, 15% off Heska lab tests, and 5-15% off Patterson dental supplies. Purchasing contracts also streamline reordering. You get consolidated ordering and billing. This saves administrative time.

Review all the vendor contracts your practice currently uses. Research where lower-cost group contracts are available. Leverage terms like no-charge freight to maximize savings. Always know your standard discount off list pricing.

The combined savings from supplier contracts can conservatively reduce a practice's expenses by 5-15%. Sign up for cooperative contracts and start saving today.

Potential Risks of Extending Client Credit

Offering payment plans or credit directly to clients may seem convenient, but it carries substantial risks that can quickly spiral out of control.

For example, just a few clients failing to pay credit balances can rapidly create major cash flow problems. This snowball effect can be financially devastating.

Failing To Utilize Industry-Specific Strategies To Optimize Cash Flow

One clinic had to lay off two staff members after multiple clients with credit accounts totaling $8,000 went delinquent. Therefore, it is generally not advisable for practices to extend credit directly to clients.

There are better financing options available that remove the risk:

✔ **CareCredit**
  ✓ This veterinary-specific payment plan from GE Capital pays your practice upfront in full. Clients repay CareCredit over 60-84 month terms at reasonable interest rates.

✔ **ScratchPay**
  ✓ Another financing option that pays practices upfront while clients repay ScratchPay over 6-12 months.

These veterinary healthcare credit cards allow clients to get financing and make payments over time without your practice taking on financial risk. You get paid immediately. Only offer direct credit in very rare cases for long-time clients with an excellent payment history. Even then, exercise extreme caution.

Many practice management software systems seamlessly integrate with CareCredit, ScratchPay, and similar services, making financing easy for both you and your clients. Leverage outside financing plans rather than put your practice at risk with in-house client credit accounts.

Tracking Key Financial Metrics

To effectively manage your practice's financial health, you need clear visibility into key metrics like:

#04 Pain Point

Failing To Utilize Industry-Specific Strategies To Optimize Cash Flow

✔ Revenue and profitability by department, doctor, and procedure

✔ Accounts receivable aging and client credit balances

✔ Inventory costs, usage, turn rates, and waste

✔ Staff salaries, benefits, and total overhead costs

✔ Revenue per veterinarian FTE

✔ Medical fee increases versus inflation

Without monitoring such metrics, it's impossible to catch financial problems early before they escalate.

Here are tips for tracking finances:

✔ Use practice management software to extract real-time financial reports. Set key benchmarks and monitor metrics over time.

✔ Review numbers at monthly management meetings. Assign action plans to address issues.

✔ Compare your metrics against industry benchmarks to identify areas for improvement. Is your revenue per doctor low?

✔ For deeper analysis, work with a veterinary accountant or advisor. Have them assess your profitability drivers.

Proactively tracking financials instead of waiting for the year-end to reconcile is vital. As the saying goes, what you measure improves. Make metrics visible to staff to drive engagement

#05
Pain Point

Not Keeping Track Of Changing Regulations So You Can Avoid Losing Your License

JENNIFER KINDRED

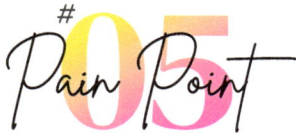

Not Keeping Track Of Changing Regulations So You Can Avoid Losing Your License

 # Pain Point 05

The veterinary industry is heavily regulated. Staying current with new laws, protocols, and compliance at the federal, state, and local levels takes significant time and resources. Failure to comply also brings major risks such as fines or loss of license.

Key regulatory areas for veterinary practices include:

✔ **Drugs**
   - ✓ The DEA and state authorities regulate the dispensing and storage of controlled substances. Proper handling and documentation are essential.

✔ **Safety**
   - ✓ OSHA oversees hazardous materials, infectious disease control, workplace injuries, and other health risks.

✔ **Disability Laws**
   - ✓ Reasonable accommodation and access for disabled clients and employees is required.
   - ✓ Medical privacy laws dictate the protection of client data and records.

✔ **Licensure**
   - ✓ Doctors and staff must maintain up-to-date licenses through continuing education and renewals.

Pain Point #05

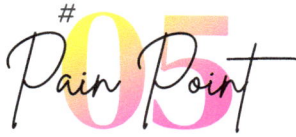

Not Keeping Track Of Changing Regulations So You Can Avoid Losing Your License

✔ Public Health

- ✓ Disease reporting and animal bite reporting may be mandatory.

- ✓ Protocols for zoonotic diseases are issued.

✔ Waste

- ✓ Medical waste disposal must follow regulations for incineration, labeling, transportation, and leak protection.

Staying compliant demands constant vigilance. Joining professional associations provides updates and guidance. Regular staff training on protocols is key. Manuals should outline all processes. A risk management assessment can identify vulnerabilities.

Leveraging technology like practice management software can aid compliance through digitized records, reminder alerts about license renewals, inventory tracking, billing controls, and data security. Outside consulting services can also review practices and recommend process improvements.

While burdensome, most regulations aim to protect public and animal health. Embracing compliance as an important responsibility of the profession can change perspectives on its challenges.

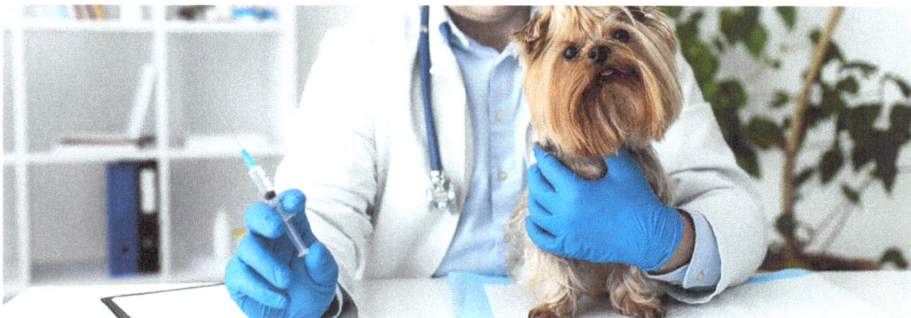

#06
Pain Point

Not Understanding The Difference Between Profit & Cash Flow So You Don't Run Out Of Cash

Pain Point

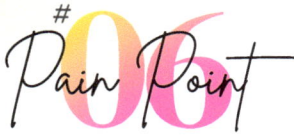

Not Understanding The Difference Between Profit & Cash Flow So You Don't Run Out Of Cash

Many veterinary practice owners struggle to properly distinguish between profit and cash flow. This lack of financial literacy can lead to poor decision-making and prevent the business from reaching its full potential.

The Key Distinctions Between Profit and Cash Flow

The key difference is that profit reflects performance on paper, while cash flow reflects the actual money moving in and out of the business. Profitability does not guarantee sufficient cash flow to pay the business owner a salary.

Real-Life Implications for Veterinary Practices

For example, a vet clinic may show $200,000 in profits last year. But if a large portion of that is still tied up in accounts receivable or inventory, the business may not have $200k readily available to distribute. The owner needs to understand cash flow levers like managing receivables, inventory, and payables cycles.

Additionally, owners should forecast and track cash flow regularly to anticipate ebbs and flows. Vet practices often experience seasonal dips in the summer or peak demand in the winter. Planning ahead and making financial decisions based on cash flow rather than profit alone will create a healthier business in the long run.

Key Takeaways for Veterinary Practice Owners

The key takeaway is that veterinary owners must learn the fundamental difference between profit and cash flow.

Pain Point #06

Not Understanding The Difference Between Profit & Cash Flow So You Don't Run Out Of Cash

This knowledge empowers them to realistically assess how much they can pay themselves while still investing back into the business.

A savvy owner does not conflate high profits with high cash flow available for distribution. Understanding this nuance is critical for the overall financial health and growth of any vet practice.

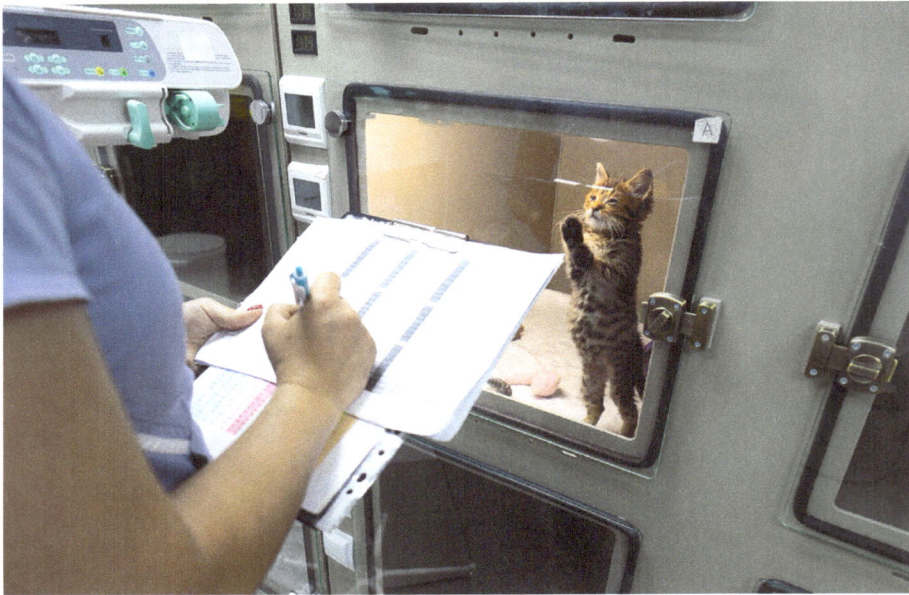

#07
Pain Point

Lack of Proper Client Communication Can Lead to the Loss of Clients

JENNIFER KINDRED

Pain Point #07

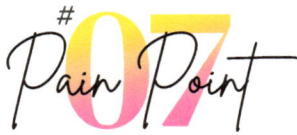

Lack of Proper Client Communication Can Lead to the Loss of Clients

Communicating effectively with clients is critical in veterinary medicine.

Educating clients about animal health management, explaining conditions, bills, and pricing, describing medical procedures, and managing care expectations all require skill. Poor communication leads to misunderstandings that damage client relationships and the practice's reputation.

Some keys for improving client communication include:

✔ **Listening**
- Let clients share information without interruption. Ask open-ended questions and show interest in their perspectives.

✔ **Clear Explanations**
- Use layman's terms to explain medical issues, procedures, aftercare instructions, and bills. Check for understanding by having clients explain back to you.

✔ **Patience and Empathy**
- Clients are emotionally invested in their pets. Anxiety, frustration, or denial influences the reception of information. Validate feelings and give space rather than reacting defensively if clients get upset.

✔ **Managing Expectations**
- Be clear upfront about possible outcomes, limitations, risks, and costs of treatments so clients have reasonable expectations.

✔ **Follow Up**
- Call or email after visits or procedures to check on pets and address any lingering client questions.

#07 Pain Point

Lack of Proper Client Communication Can Lead to the Loss of Clients

✔ **Front Desk Training**

✓ Ensure receptionists provide great customer service skills and can answer basic client questions.

Simple improvements like intake questionnaires to understand client concerns and better invoice detailing also facilitate communication. Improving skills takes practice but progress pays off in client appreciation.

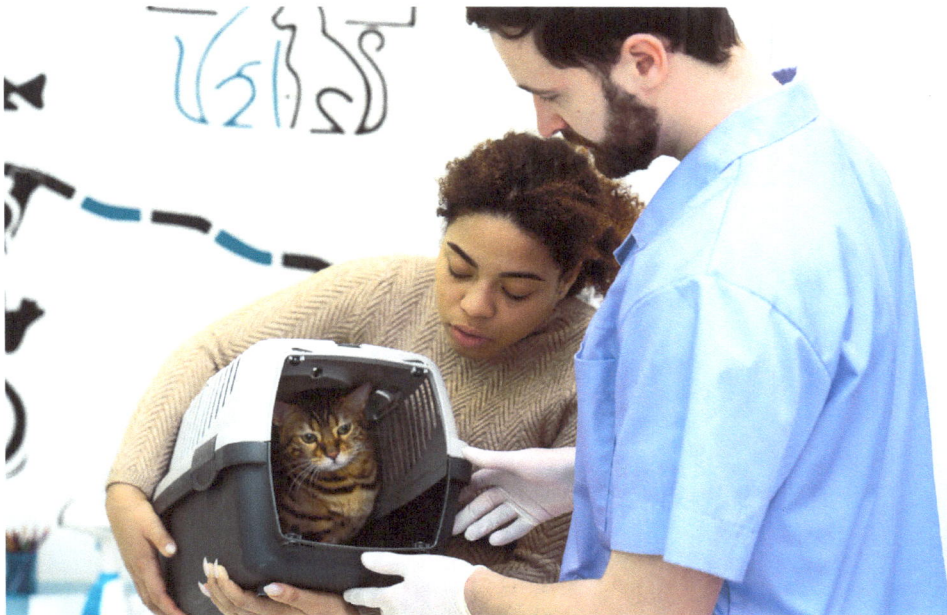

Kindred
FINANCIAL SERVICES

Pain Point #08

Failing To Practice Self Care and Time Management So You Don't Burn Out and Lose Clients

JENNIFER KINDRED

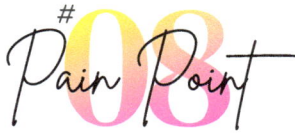

Failing To Practice Self Care and Time Management So You Don't Burn Out and Lose Clients

Veterinary medicine is extremely demanding. Long hours are standard, especially early in careers. Night and weekend on-call shifts are common. The work is physically and emotionally draining. As a result, burnout and mental health issues are very high among vets.

Achieving a better work-life balance starts with recognizing limits. The culture of self-sacrifice instilled in vet med school leads many to neglect personal needs. Set boundaries and learn to say no when overwhelmed. Also watch for signs of burnout like irritability, lack of focus, and withdrawal.

There are ways to build more personal time:

✔️ **Schedule Breaks**
   ✓ Take lunch, don't work through it. Try to leave on time some days.

✔️ **Limit On-Call**
   ✓ Negotiate a reasonable on-call schedule. Share the load if possible.

✔️ **Take Vacations**
   ✓ Use allotted funds for travel, hobbies, and recharging. Unplug from work email.

✔️ **Daily Balance**
   ✓ Make time for exercise, relationships, and activities beyond work. Say no to non-essential obligations.

✔️ **Mentors**
   ✓ Seek guidance from vets with good work-life balance on setting boundaries.

Failing To Practice Self Care and Time Management So You Don't Burn Out and Lose Clients

For business owners, foster a culture that values rest and balance. Institute PTO limits to force staff to recharge. Promote activities like staff outings or office exercise breaks. Lead by example on not overworking. The path to sustainability lies in healthier work habits.

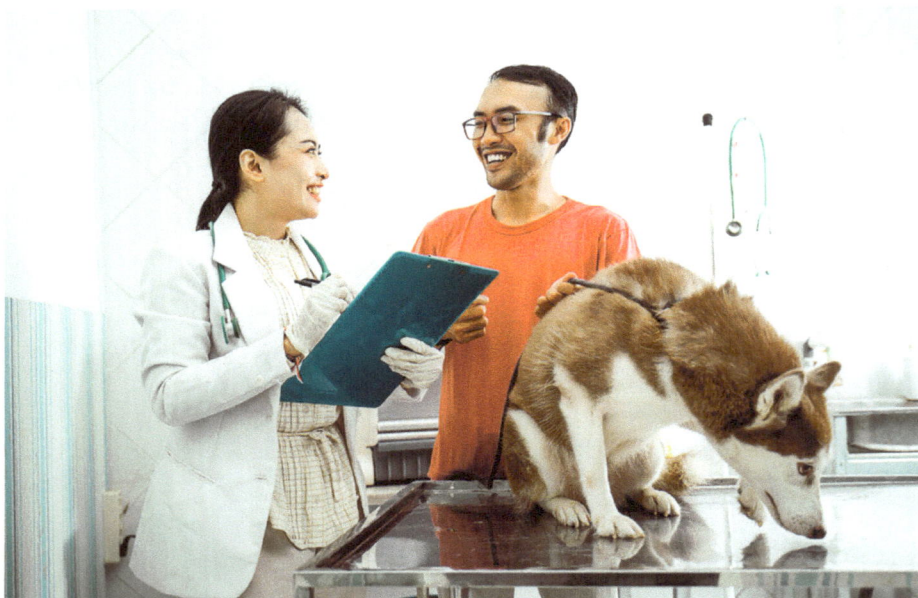

#09 *Pain Point*

Technology Deficiencies Will Hamper Productivity and Cause Organizational Challenges

JENNIFER KINDRED

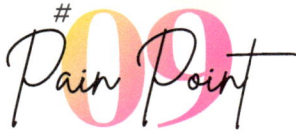

Technology Deficiencies Will Hamper Productivity and Cause Organizational Challenges

From communications to medical records to practice management, technology plays a huge role in veterinary practices.

However, clinics often suffer from outdated systems, inefficient paper workflows, and fragmented or minimally used software tools. This drives costs, hampers productivity, and creates organizational challenges.

Some common technology pitfalls include:

- ✔️ **Outdated Practice Management Software**
  - ✓ Core workflow systems haven't been updated in years, lacking modern features and mobility.

- ✔️ **Paper Medical Records**
  - ✓ Handwritten charts and prescription pads lead to filing errors, vain searches for info, and difficulty analyzing data.

- ✔️ **Client Communication**
  - ✓ Lacking client portals or two-way texting to conveniently share updates and documents. Still rely on phone calls.

- ✔️ **Inventory Management**
  - ✓ No automation of reordering and tracking. Expired products and supply shortages are common.

- ✔️ **No Integration**
  - ✓ Different applications like billing, lab results, and imaging don't sync, requiring constant manual data entry.

Pain Point #09

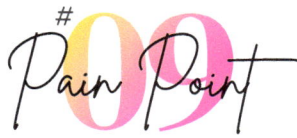

Technology Deficiencies Will Hamper Productivity and Cause Organizational Challenges

✔ Cybersecurity

✓ Weak access controls and unprotected networks risk data breaches.

Transitioning to integrated, cloud-based platforms with robust practice management, medical records, client communication, and inventory tools can transform efficiency. Training staff in optimization is key. Look for systems with veterinary-specific features and workflows.

The time and cost of upgrading technology can seem daunting but pays long-term dividends in performance, growth, and staff satisfaction from smoother operations.

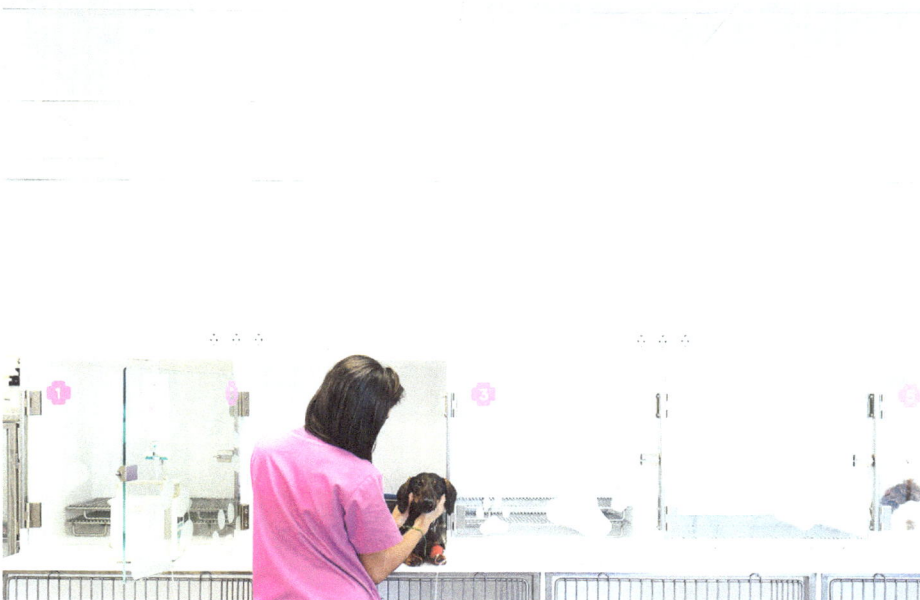

#10
Pain Point

Failing To Work With An Accounting Advisor With First Hand Knowledge From Owning Her Own Veterinary Practice

JENNIFER KINDRED

Pain Point #10

Failing To Work With An Accounting Advisor With First Hand Knowledge From Owning Her Own Veterinary Practice

Most veterinarians enter the field focused on medicine, not business management. But practice owners must master a broad set of business skills from finances and marketing to human resources. Learning these on the job while also delivering care is extremely difficult.

Common issues faced include:

✔ **Budgeting and Cash Flow**
- ✓ Many don't understand key financial indicators or properly plan cash reserves for slow periods, causing shortfalls.

✔ **Pricing Services**
- ✓ Pricing is set arbitrarily without analyzing overhead costs, market comparisons, and communicating value.

✔ **Marketing**
- ✓ Ineffective marketing fails to reach new clients beyond the existing patient base. Websites and social media are underutilized.

✔ **Staff Management**
- ✓ Hiring, training, evaluating, and retaining staff lacks consistency without human resource systems in place. Conflict resolution suffers.

✔ **Inventory Management**
- ✓ Inventory costs are too high due to overstocking, expiration, and poor tracking.

Failing To Work With An Accounting Advisor With First Hand Knowledge From Owning Her Own Veterinary Practice

☑ **Data and Technology**
  ✓ Outdated or fragmented practice software undermines efficiency, data access, and organization.

Addressing these business gaps is critical for long-term success. Steps that can help include:

☑ Taking business courses and webinars

☑ Hiring experienced practice managers

☑ Getting mentorship from successful practice owners

☑ Using veterinary-specific software tools

☑ Outsourcing specialized functions like marketing and HR

Building a supportive team and allocating time to plan and work "on" the practice, not just "in" it, is essential. The profession would also benefit from integrating more business training into the vet school curriculum.

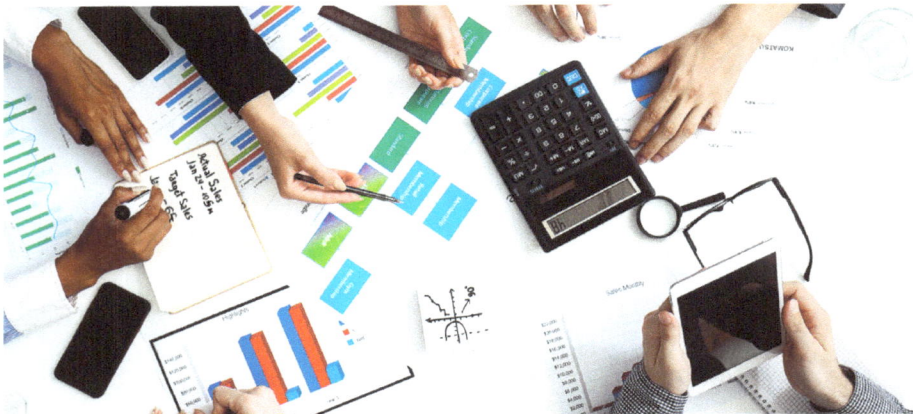

Conclusion

Would you like to increase your veterinary practice's profits and cash flow while minimizing taxes and risk?

If you read this book and realized that you may be making one of the ten costly mistakes in your business, and you feel that your mistakes are beyond repair, don't lose hope...

We specialize in helping veterinarians overcome their mistakes and plan a better future for their business. We care about the veterinary community and are here to help you.

I would like to offer you a free 30-minute consultation to see if we can implement the strategies in this guide into your business.

There is no obligation on your part, and I will not hold anything back...

By the end of our call, you will have a clear plan for what you need to do to turn your veterinary practice into a wealth-generating machine.

The best-case scenario is that I will help you save thousands of dollars and dozens of hours every year.

In the worst-case scenario, you will find out that you are not leaving any money on the table. Does that sound fair?

Hop on a call with me and I will analyze your tax strategy, business entity structure, and accounting system to ensure that you are maximizing your veterinary practice's profits and cash flow while minimizing taxes and risk.

Talk soon,

Jennifer Kindred
KINDRED FINANCIAL SERVICES